Cancer Scores a Hat Trick

To Dierdre,

Best wishes for a Happy, Healthy & Fulfilling Life!

Shaunda Muir

Cancer Scores a Hat Trick

*Lessons About Living
Life to the Fullest*

SHAWNDA MUIR

Cancer Scores a Hat Trick

Copyright © 2011 Shawnda Muir

All Rights Reserved. No part of this publication may be reproduced, stored in a retrieval system or transmitted in any form or by any means—electronic, mechanical, photocopy, recording or any other—except for brief quotations in printed reviews, without the prior permission of the author.

ISBN: 978-1-926718-22-4
Printed in Canada

Cover Design: hollyclarkedesign.com
Book Design: Charlie Livingston

Published by

Forever Books
WINNIPEG CANADA
www.foreverbooks.ca

To my dad,
may you rest in peace.

To Darryl, Justin, and Devin,
the three wonderful men in my life.

To my mom,
the rock of the family.

Acknowledgements

Thank you to my mom and dad, Isabelle and Connie Bossuyt, who introduced me to the principles of living a balanced life with family first. The farm was truly a great upbringing, teaching me many lessons that have served me well over the years.

Thank you to my husband, Darryl, and two sons, Justin and Devin, for their never-ending support during my cancer journey and their patience while I've worked on this book. Your encouragement and love means more than I can say.

Thank you to my sister Wendy Kukelko, brother Randy Bossuyt, and sister-in-law Debbie Wionzek for their listening ears and helping hands during my cancer journey. I'm not sure I could have made it through without you.

Thank you to the many family and friends who helped raise almost a quarter million dollars in the first three years for cancer research through our Shoot for the Cure campaigns. Cancer impacts everyone. Thank you for helping to find a cure.

Special thanks to my dear friend Zdenka Melnyk for her never-ending support and writing expertise, to Sharron Stockhausen for her book writing and editing assistance, and to the many friends who have encouraged and supported me along the way, including the reviewer of this book.

Anyone else who thinks they should have been included here, well, you know who you are, and thank you!

Contents

Introduction	11
Part 1 — The Journey	13
Chapter One: Cancer Scores a Hat Trick	15
Chapter Two: The Highlight Reel	25
Part 2 — Lessons Learned	59
Chapter Three: The Power of Positive Thinking	61
Chapter Four: Take Care of Yourself First	69
Chapter Five: Live Your Ideal Life	79
Know What You Want	79
Focus On What You Want	85
Get What You Want	91
Chapter Six: Daily Happiness Checklist	97
Part 3 — Epilogue	99
Chapter Seven: Live Your Life to the Fullest	101
Appendix — Your Action Guide	111
Suggested Reading	137
About the Author	139

Introduction

The year 2007 started the way any new year does—full of hope and promise. But the anticipation of a positive and happy new year lasted about six weeks. Then everything changed.

My husband was diagnosed with cancer in February. My father was diagnosed with cancer in April. I received a cancer diagnosis in August.

Cancer scored a hat trick—and it scored it on a family who had never had a personal encounter with cancer before. In hockey, a hat trick is three goals scored by one player in a game. For our hockey-loving family, this represented a different type of hat trick—three cancer diagnoses in six months.

My husband and I survived, but my father did not. In spite of the shock, the fear, and the suffering, cancer taught me many life lessons, not the least of which is how to be happy.

I began 2007 as a career woman and hockey mom. I faced the challenge of cancer three times in six months. But I knew that all of this horrific news had a purpose. There was something I was supposed to do differently with my life and cancer was the catalyst.

In February 2008, while undergoing chemotherapy treatments, I organized a community fundraiser that raised over $135,000 for cancer research. I've continued to lead this fundraiser annually, reaching nearly a quarter million dollars in the first three years.

In 2010, I left my corporate job to better align myself with my principles and priorities, including helping my husband with our family business.

But this book is not just about me. It is also about you. It is about learning how to increase your happiness, even in the face of adversity.

I wrote this book to help you learn to live a happy fulfilling life starting now. Should tragedy come to you and yours, you will be able to face the adversity, find the silver lining of the experience, and have no regrets. The rest of your life awaits you. You can survive and be happier. I'm living proof.

Part One

The Journey

Chapter One
Cancer Scores a Hat Trick

Cancer's First Score

Imagine waking up one morning thinking all is well in your world, only to learn by day's end that your husband was at the doctor's office and the diagnosis is possible testicular cancer. I've been there.

The sun started to set as I drove home from work on February 6, 2007. With the work day behind me, I turned my thoughts toward the evening activities for our family. The plan was for my husband, Darryl, to coach hockey practice for our ten-year-old son Devin while I took our twelve-year-old son Justin to his practice. Supper simmered in the crockpot and all was well—or so I thought.

Shortly after 5:00 p.m., Darryl arrived home to say he had just been at the doctor's. When he told me his news, I was stunned. Darryl had found a lump on one of his testicles and went to the urologist to follow up.

The urologist thought Darryl might have cancer.

As Darryl calmly relayed the doctor's suspicion, I looked at him in shock. My legs turned to Jell-O. There must be some mistake. Darryl was forty-two years old. He was athletic, and by most accounts, the picture of health.

Darryl had an ultrasound the next day. Surgery was scheduled for six days later on the afternoon of February 13. That day our boys went to my sister Wendy's house after school. She lived only five doors down. I told her that Darryl and I were going out for dinner and would pick the boys up in the early evening.

Darryl and I got to the hospital around noon for his surgery that was scheduled for 2:00 p.m. Unfortunately, there were delays in the operating room and his surgery was postponed.

I called my sister around 7:00 p.m. to let her know we weren't going to get back from our dinner date as early as expected. I asked her to take the phone into a separate room because I had something to tell her. Then I told her that we hadn't gone out for dinner at all, but that we were in the hospital waiting for Darryl to have surgery for what the doctors thought might be cancer.

Wendy and I both fought back tears as we made arrangements for her to take Justin and Devin home, put them to bed, and wait for us.

At 9:30 p.m., Darryl was finally brought back to the recovery room. During the surgery to remove the testicle and tumour, the surgeon also found, and repaired, a hernia in the same area. Due to the late hour and the pain he was experiencing, Darryl ended up staying at the hospital overnight. The hernia later became our cover story because we were not comfortable telling people about Darryl's cancer yet.

About a week after surgery, we went back to the surgeon's to get the pathology test results and the tumour was confirmed cancerous. Worse yet, it appeared the cancer had spread to his stomach area lymph nodes, but the doctors didn't know to what extent. It would take another six weeks to get Darryl in for a CT scan.

This was our first direct exposure to cancer in our family.

Cancer's Second Score

The month after hearing about my husband's cancer, I got the news that my father had cancer too.

On March 5, 2007, my mom took Dad to the hospital where he had a CT scan to investigate roving pains in his abdomen, back, and groin areas. The scan indicated the presence of suspicious looking cysts, which prompted the doctors to do another scan the next morning and do more tests later that week. The outcome of these tests indicated Dad needed a biopsy of the cysts, and this procedure was scheduled for March 16.

Following the surgery, Dad was in so much pain the doctors had to increase his medications, which meant he had to stay in the hospital. He started having bad reactions to the pain killers and hallucinated unmercifully. He continually tried to pull out all his intravenous lines and get out of bed. Mom had to stay with him day and night to help keep him safe.

One day when I was staying with Dad to give my mom a break, my Uncle Lorne came to visit. Unfortunately, the medications and cancer were altering Dad's usual behavior and he wasn't his normal, positive self. He demanded Uncle Lorne take him out of the hospital. Dad and Uncle Lorne had worked together on the farm for sixty years, but none of that mattered. There was nothing my uncle could do. He felt as helpless as the rest of us.

Finally, March 19 arrived and the oncologist stopped by during his rounds. All he said was Dad needed to see another oncologist who specializes in Dad's type of tumour. He booked Dad an appointment for April 2 and, thankfully, Dad was released to go home and wait.

By March 23, just the basic act of eating hurt Dad so much that we called his general practitioner to come over for a house call. But there was nothing the doctor could do. So, Mom and Dad continued to struggle at home, waiting for April 2 to arrive.

On Thursday, March 29, I went to visit my parents and told Mom about Darryl's cancer. She was surprised and saddened, and with everything going on with Dad, she was in as much shock and emotional overload as I was.

The day before Dad's appointment, Darryl, I and the boys went to Mom and Dad's for dinner. Although we tried to remain positive and cheerful as at other family gatherings, the thoughts about the next day appeared to weigh heavily on everyone's mind.

April 2 arrived and we all went to the hospital. Coincidentally, Darryl's first chemo treatment was at the same location as Dad's biopsy appointment. Darryl and I arrived at 8:45, a few minutes late for Darryl's appointment and his 8:30 a.m. pre-chemo blood work. Mom and Dad also arrived at 8:45, a few minutes early for Dad's 9:00 a.m. blood work. This was stressful and awkward, as Dad still didn't know about Darryl's cancer and we didn't want him to know, due to his long-time anxiety condition. To avoid the possibility of an upsetting explanation, Darryl hid behind various pillars so Dad wouldn't see him. This worked well until, ironically, Dad and Darryl eventually ended up being seated next to each other to have their blood drawn. In the end, though, my dad was in such pain he didn't even realize Darryl was getting his blood drawn too. Dad simply thought Darryl was there to support him with the rest of the family.

Eventually, after the doctor reviewed Dad's biopsy results and completed an array of assessments on Dad's heart, pulse, and reflexes, he stated that Dad had a very aggressive and rare form of cancer called Burkitt's Lymphoma. Dad's final prognosis was to live only four to six weeks.

And, so, within six weeks of Darryl's diagnosis, we experienced our second direct exposure to cancer.

Cancer Scores a Hat Trick

A few months later, one Saturday morning in August, I was putting on my bathing suit and felt a lump in my breast. We were at our cottage and entertaining that weekend.

I had noticed a hard spot a couple of months earlier, but with all the other stress going on, I hadn't thought much of it. I just assumed it had something to do with the hormonal changes women talk about when they reach their forties.

But this Saturday the lump felt different from what I noticed previously. There was a hard edge to the lump, which didn't make sense if it was simply hormonal changes.

Don't panic, I told myself. *What are the chances of three of us in one family being diagnosed with cancer within six months? Better chance of winning the lotto, I'm sure!*

I made a mental note to call my doctor Monday morning, then proceeded to entertain company and enjoy swimming and water sports with the kids.

On Monday morning, August 28, I called my doctor's office. There were no appointment times available, but the receptionist offered to check with the doctor anyway. She came back moments later to say the doctor would squeeze me in at 4:00 p.m.

When I arrived for the appointment, the doctor did a physical examination and told me I had to go for a mammogram as soon as possible. I thought that was odd. My last physical was the previous December when I asked her if I needed to start getting mammograms regularly since I just turned forty. I clearly remember her response.

"Oh, no," she replied. "We don't worry about any of that until you're fifty."

My mammogram was scheduled for September 4. After the year our family had with cancer, I wanted some reassurance, so I called my girlfriend. She told me that 80 percent of lumps are not cancerous.

Phewww, I thought. *This is just one of those benign lumps that give people a scare. Stay positive.*

I had my mammogram as scheduled and was told it would take a week to get the results back to the doctor. Two days later, however, at 8:00 a.m., I was at my desk at work when the phone rang.

"Shawnda," the doctor said. "I need to see you in the office today. Come anytime and I'll fit you in, and bring your husband with you."

Ok, this is definitely sounding scarier now, I thought, *but surely it can't be cancer — not a third time in six months?*

Darryl picked me up after lunch and took me to the appointment. We weren't in the doctor's office long when she said, "I can't believe I have to tell you this, but it looks like the lump is cancerous."

The dead air was deafening until, finally, Darryl said, "It's okay, Shawnda. I survived my cancer and you can survive yours too."

"How can this be?" I asked. "Three of us in six months,

especially with none of us having cancer in our family backgrounds, and I have no other risk factors? Is there some environmental issue going on here?"

The doctor responded, "No, it's just bad luck."

I thought, *There has to be more to this hat trick of cancer than bad luck.*

And there is. Cancer's hat trick changed my life and taught me how to be truly happy, even in the face of adversity. Keep reading and I'll share those lessons with you later in the book.

Chapter Two
The Hat Trick Highlight Reel

Highlight reels typically show the best or most exciting parts of an event. The Hat Trick Highlight Reel chapter doesn't follow that rule. Instead, it shows the hardest moments we experienced during the hat trick journey, and it starts with Darryl's diagnosis.

Highlights of Cancer's First Score

Hearing that Darryl's cancer had spread to his stomach and that it was going to take six weeks to get him in for a CT scan as the next diagnostic step was scary news. But just as scary was when the surgeon then recommended we take time to ensure our financial affairs were in order in case Darryl didn't survive.

Later that night we watched a movie with the boys, then went to bed emotionally exhausted. Sleep came immediately, but it didn't last. Within a couple of hours Darryl and I woke up wide-eyed and thinking about the looming death sentence we were facing. We couldn't ignore it. We had to face the worst case scenario—Darryl's dying of cancer.

Lying in bed, we talked and cried through what would happen if Darryl didn't survive and the ramifications that brought. We talked about actions like changing life insurance policies, updating our wills, revisiting our plans to renovate our cottage. Then we talked about loved ones—how would Darryl's mom react to the news her son had cancer? She'd faced almost losing him once when he was hit by a car at age nine. He spent six months in the hospital then and was told he'd likely never walk again. He'd beaten the odds and fully recovered, but his mother's health suffered.

Agonizing over all these decisions was stressful. Then the analytical side of me kicked in. We decided I'd check with our financial advisor regarding our insurance and wills. We'd talk to Darryl's mom's doctor—he would know if her medication needed adjusting before telling her the news.

The cottage renovations needed more thought. Darryl planned, even looked forward to, working on the cottage, but he didn't want the additional financial stress on the family if he didn't survive. I decided to check with my sister to see if she would be willing to buy into the cottage to provide me with cash flow to complete the renovations in the event Darryl didn't make it.

Soon after, we learned our financial affairs were in pretty good order, my sister agreed to co-own the cottage if necessary, and Darryl's mom took the news and possible ramifications better than expected.

In our meeting with the oncologist, we learned the cancer had spread to Darryl's lymph nodes in his stomach area, putting him at Stage 2. We had further consultations with the oncologist who also consulted with other medical experts, including the doctor who treated Tour de France cyclist Lance Armstrong's testicular cancer.

Darryl had some underlying medical conditions that complicated the issue, which caused some delay in finalizing the treatment plan, but eventually Darryl chose chemotherapy over radiation because chemo provided the best chance of killing the cancer everywhere. The treatment plan was finalized as three rounds of intensive chemotherapy, starting April 2. Each round was a three-week cycle where Darryl would go to the hospital for a full morning of chemo administered intravenously on days one through five, ten, and seventeen. Then repeat the cycle starting on day twenty-two.

With the treatment plan finalized, it was now time to tell the family. It was a Thursday evening and we were out for a drive with the boys. Without warning, Darryl decided it was the right time to tell them. I panicked. How could I cuddle and console them with all of us buckled up in our seats? Darryl went ahead anyway.

"Boys," he said, "you know how I had that surgery a few weeks ago…well, next week I have to go back into the hospital for a few days to get some more treatments. I'll go in every morning and then come home for the rest of the day."

"That sounds like chemo," one of the boys said.

Darryl and I looked at each other in shock.

"Yes, it is actually chemo," I replied. "So Dad may not feel well after these treatments, and we're going to have to be careful that we don't spread any germs to him."

"That sounds like cancer," the boys said, almost in unison, seeming to take it all in stride. This was a huge relief to both Darryl and me. Later we figured out that a student at their school had been going through several rounds of leukemia treatments. The school had done a great job of educating the students about cancer and how they had to help this student stay germ-free. Our sons saw him fight cancer and survive, so surely Dad would too.

All in all, Darryl survived the chemo treatment reasonably well, but there were several challenges.

The first challenge was fatigue brought on by the intensive chemo regime coupled with Darryl owning his own company and the need to continue struggling through work. We were also working on the cottage renovations by now. Some days Darryl would go to the cottage to help. However, he'd have to go for a sleep every couple of hours. At one point, Darryl was trying to shovel some gravel and had to rest after each shovelful. This was very frustrating for Darryl, but he did persevere. It took Darryl over a year after his chemo to get back to his normal energy level.

Another difficult time happened one beautiful mid-April day when Darryl and Devin were out riding their all-terrain vehicles at the cottage. They stopped part way and when Darryl took off his helmet, he saw the dreaded clumps of hair coming out. He immediately called me up at home and asked me to be ready to shave off his hair in the morning. Little did we know that eight months later he'd be doing the same thing for me.

Darryl's other side effects from chemo included extreme fatigue, continuous nausea, bad mouth sores and loss of all taste, weight gain from steroids, blisters on his feet, calcium build-up on his toe nails, and strange lines across his back that still exist today.

The chemo ended on May 31, and in early July Darryl received test results showing the cancer cells were gone and he did not need any further treatments such as radiation. And while Darryl continues to have follow-up tests every couple of months to monitor any cancer recurrence, this news was cause to celebrate. Darryl was officially cancer-free and continues to be cancer-free.

Highlights of Cancer's Second Score

April 2 arrived. After getting Darryl settled in the chemo room for his first treatment, I went to be with my mom and dad for Dad's oncologist appointment to receive his biopsy test results.

The doctor then explained that Dad's aggressive lymphoma was in his bones, as well as having several tumors in his stomach area, with the largest being the size of a fist. Dad's original prognosis was four to six months to live.

Wow, I hadn't expected this, I thought. So many questions entered my mind.

"Isn't there some chemo you can give Dad?" I asked.

"No," the doctor said. "We would have to give your dad such high doses of chemo to beat the cancer that the chemo would kill him before the cancer would."

"What do we do then?" I asked.

"Palliative care," the doctor answered. "Use steroids and pain killers to make his last few months as pain free as possible."

Other questions came. "When do we tell Dad? How will he take it? How will the next few months go? How will Mom cope?" And the questions continued.

Eventually we left the examination room and went to the nursing station to get Dad's required prescriptions. It wasn't long after, though, when the doctor called me back into his office.

"I'm sorry to tell you" he said, "but I have to change the prognosis for your dad from four to six months to four to six weeks. We just received his blood work results from earlier today and his white blood counts have skyrocketed since his blood work five weeks ago."

Four to six weeks? I thought. *How am I going to tell Mom this awful news? Are we going to tell Dad now? How will he survive it with his anxiety?*

I thanked the doctor and left to go give Mom the update. She was just about to leave the waiting room with Dad when I pulled her aside and gave her the news.

"Four to six weeks. Are you sure?" she asked.

"Yes, unfortunately, I am, Mom. I'm so sorry. What are we going to do?"

She was silent for a long moment, then said, "I'll wait a bit until he's settled down some… then I'll tell him."

I gave her a big hug and we returned to Dad. I kissed him good-bye and helped them out of the hospital before heading back to see how Darryl was doing with his chemo treatment.

Could this nightmare really be possible? I wondered as I walked to the chemo department. *Two people in my family potentially dying of cancer at the same time?*

And while I simply wanted to fall apart with sorrow, I knew I couldn't. I had to hold myself together for Darryl's sake now, who was dealing with his first chemo treatment. So I wiped away the tears, and entered Darryl's treatment room. Not only was Darryl feeling sick, he was worried about the length of my absence, my dad's test results, and how I was coping. The nightmare impacted us all.

My mom was a solid rock as she took control of Dad's situation. She quickly looked into and then decided that she was going to do palliative care for Dad at home versus having him go into a hospital. Dad reacted so poorly in hospitals that Mom couldn't bear the thought of him spending his last days there. So we started researching how to look after someone at home. One of the first steps was having the doctors make house calls.

That Wednesday, April 4, was one of the hardest times I had to go through with my dad. When I went to visit him after work, his doctor stopped by to make a house call. Dad was in bed at the time, and Mom and I entered the room as the doctor was taking his vital signs. Then the doctor said to my dad, "Connie, do you understand you have cancer?"

"Yes," my dad replied.

I started getting nervous—where was this conversation going?

The doctor continued, "Do you understand you cannot beat this cancer; you will die from it shortly?"

I looked at my mom with a look to say, "Did you know he was going to be having this conversation, because I didn't, and I'm not sure I can handle it," as tears started filling my eyes and a lump started developing in my throat.

I looked to my dad. He slowly answered, "I guess I knew it could go this way, but I hoped it wouldn't."

And I honestly can't remember what the doctor said next

because my brain must have gone into overload and shut off temporarily. The next thing I remember is the doctor leaving the room with Mom and I was left with Dad. I wanted to cry so badly, but I couldn't. I couldn't let Dad see me sad when he was the one suffering. *Keep it together. Stay positive*, I told myself and then went and sat beside my dad.

What do you say at a time like this?

Dad started the conversation. "Well, I guess this is it then. I hoped I'd have more time to be with Mom and you kids, but I guess it's not meant to be. I've already spoken to Uncle Lorne about looking after the car for Mom when it needs oil changes. And I think I've done a pretty good job in providing her enough money to live on, so, hopefully, she will be okay."

The lump in my throat was getting bigger as I tried to talk. "Yes, Dad, Mom will be fine and we'll be here to help look after her too."

He continued. "And I think I've done well in raising you three kids, as you've all turned out pretty good. I'm really going to miss everyone, including the grandkids."

The lump in my throat felt like it was going to burst as I struggled to hold back the tears. "Dad, you've done a great job in providing for everyone and raising us kids. I don't want you to worry about anything now. You just need to rest and enjoy the next while as much as you can."

Luckily, my mom came back into the room then, which diverted the conversation. Soon after, I walked the doctor out with a hundred questions in my mind. How long will my dad live? What will happen next? How will we know when the end is near? Unfortunately, the doctor didn't have any precise answers, but we were given a tremendous palliative care booklet that walks you through the stages of a person dying. The only thing the booklet can't tell you is how long each stage will take.

I then went back to see Mom and Dad and how they were doing. Thankfully, my dad seemed at peace with the news. I felt so grateful that our family, and Dad in particular at that moment, had a strong Catholic faith. Dad did not fear death. He was sad to be leaving his loved ones on earth, but he knew he was going to a better place in heaven to be with his father Archie.

My mom and I took solace in Dad's peaceful disposition and tried remaining positive and upbeat with him. We spoke about Mom's birthday party coming up and who Dad would like to invite over. Eventually, I hugged and kissed them both good-bye and left to go check on my family, including Darryl, who had just completed his third day of chemo and was already experiencing nausea and weakness.

The next emotional challenge was Dad's final few days. Following a couple of weeks of feeling somewhat better, and socializing with friends and family, Dad went downhill quickly. Saturday, April 21, he stopped eating; Sunday he stopped drinking and talking; and on Wednesday morning, he passed away. Ironically, this was the first day of Darryl's second set of chemo treatments.

The hardest moments for me were giving Dad permission to let go and getting the phone call that the end was near.

Our priest advised us that often people dying will cling to life until a certain event happens or they have been comforted that everyone will be okay without them. It's time for them to end the pain. In my dad's case, we all took turns giving Dad this permission on the Sunday before he passed away. Dad was in a semi-conscious state at this point. After I finished speaking to him and reading him a letter from our family listing all the things we loved about him, he simply squeezed my hand and fell back asleep. I left the room fighting tears once again.

On Tuesday, the night before he passed away, all of a

sudden Dad lay quite still in his bed. He was no longer tossing in pain; rather he laid on his back with his hands at his side. We did not even give him any pain medication that night. It appeared the end was getting close. I told my mom when I left that night to call me anytime, as I did not want her being alone with my dad when he passed away. She called me at 3:00 a.m. I remember being scared when driving to their place, not sure what to expect. When I arrived, my dad's breathing was labored. Then his limbs started getting cold due to his heart not circulating the blood properly anymore. Soon his breathing became shallow, he took a few last gasps of breath, and he passed on to a greater place.

While it is sad thinking about those times, because we miss him still, it is reassuring knowing he did not suffer at the end, and now he is in a place free from suffering and pain.

Dad died on April 25, 2007, just three days before my mom's sixty-fifth birthday. The funeral was on April 27. It was held in the afternoon to allow Darryl time to complete his chemo treatment in the morning.

Highlights of Cancer's Third Score

The first challenge of my journey was waiting five weeks for lumpectomy surgery following the core biopsy, which had confirmed the tumour was cancerous.

It was hard to stay positive knowing cancer was continuing to grow inside my body while I waited. Unfortunately, I did not control the surgeon's surgery schedule and her list of more critical patients. So I tried to remain patient and positive.

In the meantime, there were other people who needed attention, starting with telling our boys the news about their mom's cancer.

It's been said that only a friend will tell you the hard truth. I'm thankful I had such a friend who warned me the boys may not take my cancer as well as they did their dad's because Mom, the rock of the family, wasn't supposed to get sick. Fortified with that wisdom, Darryl and I called the boys to us when they got home from school.

"Boys," Darryl said, "we have another family health issue we need to discuss."

"Your cancer hasn't come back, has it?"

"No, I'm fine, but someone else in the family has cancer."

"Who? Is it Granny, Grampa, Aunty, or Uncle?"

"No," Darryl said.

"Well, who else is there?" And then they looked at each other, then at me, and in unison said, "Not Mom!"

As long as I live I shall never forget that moment. "Yes, actually, it is," I said.

"Is it breast cancer?" my younger son blurted out.

"It is," I said and he put his head down and started to cry. I put my arms around them and said, "Don't worry, boys. Just as Dad had one of the most curable types of cancer for a man to get, and he survived his, so is Mom's cancer one of the most curable for a woman and I'll survive mine."

And from that moment on we remained positive every step of the way.

Next was telling my mom and sister about my news. Probably the hardest thing for my mom to deal with, beyond Dad dying, was hearing that one of her children also had cancer. Life was not supposed to work that way. The parents' role is to love and protect their children; they should not have to watch them suffer. How do I softly break my news to her?

After I told Mom and Wendy my news, we all did our best to remain strong. Mom said she wished she were the one with the cancer this time, not me. While I totally understood her feelings, being a mom myself, I told her it was okay. I was young, strong and going to beat it.

Cancer had no chance against me.

Eventually I had the lumpectomy and a couple of weeks later I received the pathology results. I had an aggressive type of cancer (insitu and invasive ductal and lobular carcinoma; the tumour was two centimeters in size, stage 2, grade 3 out of 3 on the Nottingham scale), the cancer had spread to one lymph node, was estrogen receptor positive, and HER-2 positive.

That was a lot of information to absorb. The bottom line was that I had an aggressive form of cancer, which fortunately had been caught early. The prescribed treatment plan was also aggressive and I was given an estimated five-year survival rate of over 80 percent.

My treatment plan was:

1. **Lumpectomy** surgery to remove the tumour as the primary treatment. The following treatments were secondary to help prevent a recurrence.

2. **Chemotherapy** which works on the whole body to kill off any remaining cancer cells that may have been left behind or escaped from the breast area. The drugs included FEC (Fluorouracil, Epirubicin, and Cyclophosphamide) and Taxotere administered once every three weeks for a total of six treatments.

3. **Radiation** to the area in the breast where the cancer was found. This treatment was administered daily for six weeks.

4. **Herceptin** injections to slow or stop the growth of the HER-2 protein that I tested positive for.[1] This drug was administered once every three weeks for one year.

5. **Tamoxifen** to block the effects of the estrogen hormone in the breast. This oral medication needs to be taken daily for five years.

While my treatments went fairly well there were definitely challenges along the way.

Almost all breast cancer patients will say that the waiting for the surgeries, results, and treatment plan are the hardest part. The lack of control is unsettling. I was no different, especially being someone who was used to being in charge of situations. This was the start of my learning how to adjust when you don't have control over all the variables in your life.

The next challenge was preparing for the lumpectomy. I was instructed to go to the hospital for the radioactive

---

[1] Herceptin is used to treat tumours that make too much HER-2 protein. This protein makes cancer cells grow and multiply. Herceptin attacks these cells and also alerts the immune system to destroy them. Unlike chemotherapy, which destroys all fast-growing cells, this drug only attacks the cancer cells.

injection needed for the sentinel lymph node analysis.[2] My sister-in-law, Debbie, offered to come with me because Darryl was busy with work. That was the beginning of a new routine—Debbie attending key appointments with me while Darryl focused on his work and the kids.

We were sitting outside the doctor's office when they called me in. As I got up, they called Debbie to come in too.

Okay, I thought, *If they want her to witness this procedure, I guess I am okay with that.*

Well, little did I know she would have a huge role to play. They told her to hold onto my hand while they gave me five needles around the breast area. The doctor asked if we were ready and injected the first needle of liquid into my breast tissue.

Holy Smokes! Did that hurt! I hadn't squeezed someone's hand that hard since going through thirty-two hours of labour with my first son and squeezing Darryl's hand so hard that I bent his wedding ring.

Debbie was caught off guard as well; neither of us was prepared for the pain—and then they had to repeat it four more times. Darryl was lucky he missed that

---

2 Removal and examination of the first sentinel lymph node to which cancer cells are likely to spread from a primary tumor.

appointment, although apparently the procedure is not that painful for all patients.

Later during the lumpectomy, the doctor had to remove all the lymph nodes under my arm (fourteen), as the first sentinel lymph node had tested positive for cancer. The result was that the surgery took longer than expected — worrying Darryl and Debbie who were pacing in the waiting room. I had to have a drainage bag attached to my side for two weeks, as well as experiencing long-term numbness and risk of lymphedema (swelling of the arm).

Before chemo could start, I went for day surgery to have a port[3] put under my chest skin to help facilitate the many needles and injections I'd be having over the next year and a half. While having this surgery was a little unsettling, it was nothing compared to when they had to remove the port almost two years later, due to all the tissue having grown around it.

The side effects of the chemo started almost immediately. The evening before the treatment, I took steroids which were supposed to help reduce the side effects of the chemo. Unfortunately, the steroids kept me awake at night and then inevitably worrying about the next day's events.

---

3 A port is an implanted device through which blood may be withdrawn and drugs may be infused without repeated needle sticks.

Next, I had to endure the treatment itself. I would go to the hospital and have the chemo drugs injected via an intravenous line into my port. For some drugs, I needed to chew on ice and suck popsicles to freeze my mouth. This helped minimize the amount of blood and thus chemo going into my mouth, which in turn helped reduce the number of mouth sores and blisters later. Other drugs would make me feel severely chilled, so I'd wrap myself in heated blankets.

Shortly after arriving home from the first three treatments of chemo (FEC), I would get nauseous and start vomiting. I'd feel fatigued and be in a "brain fog" where it was hard to think straight, or get motivated to do anything. This was especially challenging for me, the person with a mile long to do list. Finally on day four, the side effects would lighten up and I'd start feeling better. The side effects from chemo treatments four through six (Taxotere) were primarily achy muscles and joints and my finger nails becoming loose.

Three weeks after my first chemo treatment the dreaded moment happened—my hair started coming out in clumps in the shower. As much as I tried to prepare myself for that moment, it was still hard since it was visible proof that I was a cancer patient. I called out to Darryl, had a cry on his shoulder and then asked him to shave my head, just as I had done for him eight months earlier.

Another challenge was that my white blood counts were not recovering quickly enough after each chemo treatment, causing the following treatment to be delayed. These delays were very difficult for me, an organizer, as I had my winter planned out, based on the anticipated chemo dates.

Since my white counts continued to be low, I had to learn how to give myself Neupogen injections (a white blood cell booster), which I needed to take on days five through ten following the chemo treatment. This was difficult since normally I am uncomfortable with even the sight of needles, let alone administering them to myself regularly. Nevertheless, I did fairly well for the first two sessions.

However, when it came to the third round, I didn't fare as well. Day five arrived and I was set to start giving myself the dreaded injections for the coming week. It was a Monday morning. The kids were getting ready for school and Darryl was having breakfast with us, which was unusual given his normal morning schedule—but very lucky for me.

I was sitting in our breakfast nook on the bar stool. I asked Darryl to get me the medicine kit from the fridge. As I was pulling out the needle and Neupogen liquid, I started feeling ill. *This is strange,* I thought. *I don't normally get sick this long after the chemo.* Then it got worse.

Feeling the urge to vomit, I called out, "Devin, can you get me a bucket please? I think I'm going to throw up."

Soon after, I announced, "Here it comes," and the next thing I knew I was waking up on the floor, staring at the ceiling, with a panicked Darryl leaning over me. Apparently after saying, "Here it comes," my eyes rolled back in my head, my arms went up, and I started falling backwards off the bar stool.

Darryl had been keeping an eye on me, and when he saw me starting to fall backwards, he lunged out to catch me before I hit the table behind me and the floor. I was out cold for probably half a minute, although Darryl said it seemed much longer, as he was panicking and calling out to the kids to come help.

As I started coming to, I tried to sit up. But it was not to be. I was way too weak, so I promptly lay down again on the kitchen floor. I asked the kids to bring me a pillow and blanket, and stayed there for over half an hour before finally getting enough strength to get up.

Later the doctors determined that I had likely fainted because of getting too worked up about the upcoming needles. From then on, I ensured I was sitting on a couch in a safe setting when giving myself injections.

My radiation treatments were quite short in duration—

approximately fifteen minutes each. However, fatigue was a major side effect. I'm not sure if it was primarily from the treatment itself, or the hassle of getting to and from the appointment every day. But the bottom line was I needed to allow myself time to get extra rest during these treatments.

As I anticipated, physically, the cancer was challenging to overcome but I did persevere. Little did I know that the mental aspect of the cancer journey would be even more challenging for me and last a lot longer than the physical recovery.

I learned that the return to normal life after cancer treatments is one of the hardest challenges for many patients. The doctors, and books about cancer, say that often patients go into varying stages of depression following the completion of their treatments. There are several reasons for this.

- The support network of doctors and nurses is no longer available to them on a daily basis. While you are getting your treatments, you feel safe and are sure the medical staff will quickly catch any problems that may arise. Who will be looking out for your well-being now?

- They have expectations from other people as well as themselves now that they are supposed to be back to normal (i.e., the many tasks around the house that have slipped over the treatment period, and reintegrating back into their work if they took a leave). However, research shows that cancer patients are not fully recovered until at least three times the length of their treatments. For example, if your chemo and radiation took six months, then you are not back to your normal self for at least a year and a half.

- Virtually all cancer patients go through a period of self-reflection during their journey, and vow to make changes in their lives. But it takes a lot of willpower to actually follow through with these commitments and not slip back to the old routines prior to cancer, especially when life gets busy again.

When cancer scored its hat trick on our family, I also went through a period of self-reflection. I wondered why our family got hit with three cancer diagnoses in such a short time and what I was supposed to do about it.

When Darryl was first diagnosed, we told ourselves that everyone has a chance of getting cancer. It was Darryl's unlucky turn. So deal with it and move on. Then with my dad's diagnosis, even though he was only seventy-four years old, he did have Parkinson's disease and was dreading a slow, debilitating death, so his quick departure from suffering was a partial blessing in disguise. But when I was diagnosed, I couldn't help but wonder why? What message about life from up above was I just not getting?

Before cancer, my job was the director of a product line in a large insurance company, heading up a major claims/IT project. I was a wife and mother of two energetic pre-teen boys. I was the office administrator/bookkeeper for my husband's construction business. And I was an active member of the community. Reflecting back, I was definitely stretching the principle of living a balanced life that my parents had taught me.

During my cancer treatments, one of the books I read was Steven Covey's *7 Habits of Highly Effective People*. Habit #2—Begin with the End in Mind was particularly relevant at this time in my journey. It posed questions such as "What do you enjoy spending time on?" My answer was leadership and wellness. "What is your purpose in life?" I knew my purpose was helping others. "What is the one thing in life that you've always feared but would like to conquer?" My response was public speaking. Interestingly, none of my answers fit well anymore with my current line of work.

During the summer, I continued reading my wellness and personal development books with vigour. I was also preparing for an upcoming speech I had been asked to give by a friend for her company on our family's experience with cancer. This was exciting, as it was my first opportunity to test out my dream of helping others through public speaking. It went over well, with audience members encouraging me to do more inspirational speaking.

Once I had recovered from my treatments, my return-to-work date was tentatively scheduled for October 15, one year following my surgery. However, this is where the work challenges started. Someone else had been placed in my old position during my absence to take over the project I was leading, which made sense. But where did that leave me now? At one point, my employer considered offering me a wellness director position in the company. This role would have potentially been a perfect fit for my passions, but it fell through due to timing and budgets. Eventually they outlined a different role, which changed to another, with continued delays happening during each step. While I understood it was a challenge for my employer to find me an appropriate position, the delays and uncertainty were also very stressful for me.

My cancer councillor summed it up well, "You cannot get on with your life and close the cancer chapter until all parts of your life are back together—including your work."

At one point I considered leaving my job, but my councillor strongly suggested that it would not be a good idea to make a major career change in the midst of my full physical recovery and emotionally distraught state.

So I continued practising my daily mantra, telling myself to be patient and positive. I could not control my job situation, but I could control my behaviour and thoughts.

My return to work was finally scheduled for January 4, 2009. I was assigned to a project for a year. Unfortunately, a short while later the project started to fizzle and my role dwindled, along with my self-confidence. As most people, I wanted to feel like I was contributing and adding value at work. Be patient and positive, I kept telling myself. My employer assured me that by summer a re-organization would take place and I would be integrated back into a meaningful role.

Fortunately at that time, I discovered the "Don't Sweat the Small Stuff" series by Richard Carlson. It includes books on learning how to deal with work, home, family, etc. by bringing more peace, love, and kindness into your life. I read these books every day, listened to the audio, and eventually started learning how to apply the lessons on a daily basis. I was slowly regaining control of my happiness—even when I couldn't control all the variables, such as my work. Learning this was a *major* lesson for me, the person who usually thrives on being in control.

Summer arrived and not much was happening on the work front—it was pretty slow and unfulfilling. So I tried focusing on all the positives. Because work wasn't too demanding, I was able to get away for my summer holidays without difficulty. And I had a great time at the cottage with the family. I had finished my year of Herceptin injections without any major complications. Darryl and I continued to be cancer free, which was a huge reason to celebrate every day.

Back on the work front, the delays to a meaningful role continued until December when I finally was moved back to my old department with my staff. I was hopeful that soon I could close the cancer chapter of my life.

The new year 2010 started off fairly well. It felt great to be back with my staff. Over the next few months, though, it became apparent that the old feelings of satisfaction and fulfillment in my career weren't there anymore.

Before I knew it, the fall season arrived, with its increased pace of life both at work and at home.

I started driving the kids to school, which meant I had to drop them off before going to work and rush to pick them up at the end of the day before the school closed. And the kids' hockey seasons were starting. That usually meant challenges at the beginning of the season until the teams were all picked and settled. This year was no different.

I had a couple more speeches to give in mid-October (breast cancer awareness month) that were exciting, yet time consuming to prepare. Part of my speech included talking about some profound words of advice I received from a cancer doctor when my radiation was completed. He spoke about the importance of living your life in such a way that should cancer come back, you will have no regrets. This includes carrying out your dreams now, versus putting things off into the future.

I told the audience that writing a book about my journey was something I dreamed of doing. Some members of the audience then called me to task. Are you working on your book now, and if not, why not? Good question. When could I fit that into my hectic life right now?

Soon after, I was asked to consider speaking at the 2011 World Conference on Breast Cancer in Hamilton, Ontario in June 2011. My first reaction was, *Wow, that would be so exciting and rewarding.* But then my second reaction was, *How was I ever going to fit that in to my already over-booked schedule?*

At this time, Darryl's company was doing well and growing which was very satisfying for him. However, the more work contracts he took on, the more administration and bookkeeping I had to do. Usually I did this work from 10:00 p.m. to midnight and on weekends in between the kids' hockey games.

I survived each hectic week by telling myself I'd get caught up on the weekend. Sunday night would arrive, though, I'd see all the work still left and, with disillusionment, realize I had to go back to my corporate job the next day. *How and when was I ever going to get caught up? This doesn't seem like my vision of a balanced life. Patient and positive,* I reminded myself. *Keep pushing, slowly but surely. Which nights this week could I fit some extra work in?*

One Monday night in late fall, I was talking to my sister-in-law Debbie about how tired I was—not just physically, but tired of pushing myself so hard all the time.

Debbie reminded me, "You're falling into your trap again that you vowed you wouldn't following cancer. You're getting to bed too late every day and getting too little sleep."

"I know, I know," I replied sullenly. "I need to change something."

"What are your options?" Debbie asked.

"Well, my health is my first priority, which includes

slowing down. Second is my family. I'm not willing to give up any of my time with them. Third is helping Darryl with his company, as owning our own company has always been a dream of ours together. Fourth, is finding a way to live my passions, which is leadership and wellness, and helping others to be happier and healthier. Fifth is my corporate job."

"How do you feel about your corporate job?"

"That's a tough one," I answered. "I've been working at this company for almost eighteen years, and before cancer never would have imagined leaving until my retirement. Since cancer, though, the job is just not the same. My role has changed; my interests, passions, and priorities have changed. And while the job was definitely much better this past year than in my first year returning from cancer, it is no longer fulfilling. And as much as I find ways to remain positive every day and focus on the silver linings along the way, it uses up a lot of energy trying to remain positive when there is no longer a fit."

"On the other hand, the job does provide a healthy pay cheque, which contributes to my family's current standard of living. I don't think I can leave if it will create family financial stress."

So I sadly concluded, "I don't think I have an option at this point other than to let go of my passions—at least for a while until the kids are older and finished school."

Later that night I was doing Darryl's company work when all of a sudden I had an epiphany. I realized that with the additional work Darryl had taken on, there was enough profit in the company that I could be taking out a pay cheque for myself. Based on our monthly budget, the combination of Darryl's and my salary from his company would be enough to cover our expenses. While we wouldn't have as much discretionary income as we did with my work salary and benefits, we could maintain our current standard of living.

As soon as I realized we did not *need* my salary, I knew what change I had to make. Going back to the doctor's profound words, "live your life in such a way that should the cancer come back you will have no regrets," I no longer had a choice. If I continued pushing myself at the daily pace I was and the cancer did come back, I would always regret it. Now that I knew I did not *need* to stay at work, if I did stay, I'd feel like I contributed to the cancer's return by not taking care of myself as well as I could have.

All the stars were finally aligning and the answer to my questions—"Why? What message from up above was I just not getting?" was becoming clear. Cancer was the catalyst I needed to make a significant change in my life to more closely align with my principle of living a balanced life and my priorities—my health, my family, our family business, and my passions. I needed to "retire" from my corporate job.

Whereas I earlier couldn't imagine ever leaving work and was scared at the thought of leaving my pay cheque, benefits, and pension, now that decision simply felt right.

Darryl was in full support, "I always knew it would come down to this, but you had to be the one to make the decision when the timing was right. I'm proud of you!"

December 17, 2010, was my last day at my corporate job.

There you have it, the highlight reel from cancer's hat trick. Some of the events were hard to experience. Others were easier. But all of them helped shape our life today. We learned a lot from cancer's triple blow. The next section shares those lessons with you.

Part Two

Lessons Learned

Chapter Three
The Power of Positive Thinking

At some point, many cancer survivors will tell you that being diagnosed with cancer was the best thing that ever happened to them. I'm not sure I agree the cancer diagnosis is the best thing that ever happened to me, but it ranks right up there with marrying Darryl and being Mom to Justin and Devin. I've learned more about living a happy and fulfilling life since cancer invaded my life than I learned my entire lifetime before.

One of the best lessons I learned through my cancer experience is how powerful positive thinking is. When I focused on the positive, I felt better, I had less stress, and I could see more possibilities. Remember my revelation about leaving my corporate job to honor my passion and priorities? Positive thinking allowed me to see that possibility instead of just thinking I couldn't do it.

Cancer challenged us on many levels. While there were many challenges through Darryl's diagnosis, there were also many positives.

- Owning a general construction business, Darryl had clients and sub-trades to consider. The clients were very understanding, and the sub-trades all pitched in to help out so Darryl wouldn't lose any business.

- On his first day of chemo, Darryl met Ken, another testicular cancer patient, and they've become good friends and spend many great times fishing together now—both appreciating each day that they have.

- Darryl maintained a positive attitude throughout all his diagnosis and treatments, which was a huge benefit for the family. I remember when he first told me about the cancer and I was in shock, I got my strength from following his calm and positive lead—"Let's not worry until we know anything for sure." And that's how we've treated every hurdle we've faced along the way. Think positive until proven otherwise.

- Darryl did an awesome job renovating our cottage, which was his primary distraction to keep him motivated through his treatments.

Lessons Learned

When first reading my dad's story, you might not think there were many positives that came from his experience, but you'd be wrong. There were positives to share.

- My dad had been diagnosed with Parkinson's disease several years earlier, which is a progressive and debilitating disease. My dad was terrified of becoming incapacitated while dying a slow death. He always said he wished he would die of a heart attack at night when the time was right. So in the end, the cancer allowed him to have a quick death without a lot of suffering.

- My dad had the best farewell one could ask for. While dad had been in significant pain in the hospital during March, following the diagnosis, the doctor prescribed some steroid medication that shrunk the tumours and actually reduced the pain for him. Since he loved to socialize, this allowed us to organize several large gatherings with family and friends for people to say good-bye.

- I experienced for the first time, someone's final breaths on earth and passing on to heaven. This was one of the most peaceful events I have ever witnessed, as Dad was no longer suffering in pain.

While my diagnosis brought challenges, they were far out-weighed by the many positives during that year.

- The first highlight was the cancer fundraiser called "Shoot for the Cure" that I put on while in the midst of my chemo. "Shoot for the Cure" was a grassroots hockey and ringette campaign in my community, aimed at increasing knowledge about cancer, raising money for cancer research, and getting the community involved in a good cause. It was a tremendous success raising over $135,000 the first year. Just as importantly, it was a great coping mechanism for me, as it gave me something positive to focus on to take my mind off all my treatments. "Shoot for the Cure" has reached nearly a quarter million dollars in the first three years.

- Another huge positive that occurred during my cancer journey was the time off from work which provided more time with my kids. For the first time in their lives, I was home to see them before school and often at lunch time. And that summer, I was able to spend the full two months with them at the lake. I really enjoyed the slower pace and more balanced living. In many ways, this year off from work was the best year of my life.

- Finally, time to discover myself. I view the cancer year as a gift since it gave me an opportunity to dwell on what really is my purpose in life, my passions, my priorities, and whether I was spending my time appropriately.

Having a positive attitude was definitely a huge contributor to my cancer hat trick survival. But I don't want to limit positive thinking to dealing with catastrophic health issues. It's also a critical factor to facing whatever challenges life throws at us—family problems, career decisions, tragedies. Even daily issues that seem small, like a traffic jam, can build into stressful moments.

In her book, *The How of Happiness*[1], Sonja Lyubomirsky states that people's happiness levels are determined as follows:

- Fifty percent is based on your set point—what you were born with, your genes.

- Ten percent comes from life circumstances such as whether you are rich or poor, healthy or unhealthy.

- Forty percent is intentional activity such as attitude and behaviour.

That's great news because while you can't control your genes or many of your life circumstances, you can control at least 40 percent of your happiness.

How do you do this? You can learn it, as I did. Following

---

1 Lyubomirsky, Sonya. *The How of Happiness*. New York: Penguin Press, 2008.

are some of the main coping mechanisms I used during my cancer journey.

Determine the worst case scenario, decide how you would handle it, then focus on the best case scenario. We used this technique in the early stages of Darryl's diagnosis. Darryl dying would be the worst case scenario. We determined back up plans for how I'd handle key components of life should this happen, but then we put the worst case out of our mind and focused on the best case—him living. During my decision to leave work, we discussed what would be the worst case scenario—we lose our revenue stream from Darryl's company. How would we handle it—we'd go look for other jobs. We are both employable, so that would not be the end of the world. Then we focused on the best case scenario—Darryl's company continuing to thrive, and me achieving a better balance in life while following my principles, priorities, and passions.

Look for the silver lining in every situation. My cancer provided me a year off work with pay and extra time to strengthen my relationship with my boys. And on days when my boys would frustrate me, I'd remind myself that I am fortunate to have children at all.

Focus on the glass being half full, not half empty. I focused on the days I spent at the cottage with my family instead of the days I spent in the hospital having treatment.

Find something positive to focus on. Darryl looked forward to the cottage renovations. I looked forward to the fundraiser, Shoot for the Cure, I started. Whatever it is you're focused on doesn't have to be big—it just has to be something positive that you're excited about.

Surround yourself with positive people. We had family, friends, other cancer survivors, councillors, and I had the Shoot for the Cure community. Reach out to people around you who are supportive and positive.

Look for the lessons to be learned from every situation. Every challenge offers a positive lesson. I learned to slow down in life, to accept that I cannot control everything, to appreciate each moment, and that the small stuff isn't worth stressing over.

Be grateful. My gratitude list is huge. It includes my survival, ongoing good health, friends, fundraiser success, beautiful cottage, and on and on. I'm sure your list is huge too. Go ahead and start making it and you'll feel the good, positive feelings grow within you.

Perform an act of kindness. One thing that works for me when I'm feeling down is to think of something I can do to make someone else feel better. It's selfish in a way because when they feel better, I do too. It doesn't have to be anything big or expensive. For example, I've given family members a back massage or a foot soak. Sometimes I bake cookies. Sometimes I just open a door for someone or smile at a stranger, or let another car into the lane ahead of me. It all counts.

Read books that inspire you. I'm sure you can find books that make you feel good, give you hope, make you think "what if?", and make you glad to be alive. Read them. Enjoy them. Give yourself the gift of inspiration.

You can control your happiness, even in the face of adversity. And you can do it starting right now.

Chapter Four
Take Care of Yourself First

This lesson—taking care of yourself first—may be the most difficult one to learn because most likely you, like me, previously focused on caring for everyone else first. We make sure our families are taken care of, our customers are taken care of, our co-workers have what they need from us, etc. If (and that's a big if) there's any time or energy left over for us, we take it, but may feel a bit guilty or selfish.

That stops now. You need to take care of yourself first so you can take care of others. If your car runs out of gas, it can't do its job of moving you from place to place. If you face a serious health issue like cancer, you can't ignore it and expect to recover. Just as you need to add fuel to the car so it can function again, you need to follow your treatment plan so you can reclaim your life.

At a cancer retreat I attended, a doctor asked, "How many of you are religious about taking your chemo medicine on a regular basis?" Of course, all our hands went up. Then he asked, "How many of you are just as dedicated about getting your exercise, sleep, eating well, and looking after yourself mentally, emotionally, and spiritually?" The hands went down.

I got his message, and so did the rest of the group. Proactively taking care of ourselves is just as important in preventing cancer from returning as taking our medicine was.

According to *Canadian Cancer Statistics 2010*[1], women will be diagnosed with 48 percent and men with 52 percent of new cancer cases each year at the time of the writing of this book. While more men than women are diagnosed with cancer historically, the gap between the two has narrowed. There is good news, however. Cancer survival rates are increasing every day. And up to half of all cancers can be avoided by introducing fundamental changes in your lifestyle.

According to CancerCare Manitoba, here are some specific changes you can incorporate to help prevent cancer:

- Shape up—Get exercise every day. It's as easy as a ten minute walk three times a day.

- Eat well—Follow the Canada Food Guide, includ-

---

[1] Canadian Cancer Society's Steering Committee: Canadian Cancer Statistics 2010. Toronto: Canadian Cancer Society, 2010.

ing lots of fruits and vegetables and several glasses of water every day. Limit alcohol intake.

- Be tobacco free—If you don't smoke, don't start. If you do smoke, do everything you can to stop, and avoid second-hand smoke.

- Cover up—Protect yourself from the sun and check your skin regularly for any changes.

- Check up—Follow cancer screening guidelines and report health changes to your doctor or dentist. Early detection is another critical way you can increase your odds of beating cancer if you're diagnosed.

Before my diagnosis, I did a fairly good job of taking care of myself, but I usually came after everyone else. Cancer taught me what the airlines have been telling us for years—take care of yourself first so you can take care of others (the airlines tell us to put on our own oxygen masks before helping someone else in an emergency). If I didn't take care of myself first, I would not survive my cancer treatments to be around to take care of my family in the long run. Now I put my own health in front of the many family and work obligations that used to take priority. I've even learned to take afternoon naps without feeling guilty.

So, how do you start taking care of yourself? Begin by looking at the four dimensions of your body—physical, mental, emotional, spiritual. You need to acknowledge and embrace each one. We may think we can do three out of four and everything will work out, but the truth is that if we ignore just one of these dimensions, the other three suffer.

Physical (body)

This dimension includes exercise, nutrition, sleeping well, and stress management. Most people are aware of the need to exercise and eat healthy foods. They may not do either one well or consistently, but they know they should. Too often, however, people don't realize how important it is to get enough sleep or to manage their stress level.

Adults require between seven and nine hours of sleep every day. Since each of us is different, we need to determine how much sleep we need individually. Become aware of your body's natural sleep cycle (when you prefer to go to bed, when you awaken, etc.). If it takes you more than twenty minutes to fall asleep, get up and do something else for a little while (just make sure that something is not too stimulating).

Take naps if you like, but limit your nap to less than an

hour. Some experts say taking a ten-minute nap during the afternoon will buy you an extra hour of productive time in the evening. The point is you want to make sure you get enough sleep.

We all have stress in our lives, but not all stress is bad. Eustress is a type of stress that is fun and exciting and is good for us. Some people like racing to meet a deadline. Others like the stress of skiing down a mountain.

Acute stress is a short-term stress that can be either good or bad. We deal with acute stress every day and some excites us while other stress frustrates us.

Chronic stress seems to go on and on without end. We can't seem to escape it and it eventually wears us down. There are many possible sources of chronic stress, including challenging children, bad marriages, unsatisfactory jobs, busy lives, etc. Too much chronic stress can trigger physical symptoms, and it's been estimated that the majority of doctors' visits are symptoms that are partially stress-related. So be aware of the stress in your life and its impact on you physically.

While I didn't think I was an overly stressed person before cancer, I did know I was on the borderline due to my hectic lifestyle. And I wonder if stress did play a part in my cancer diagnosis, as I had none of the usual risk factors for breast cancer.

Stop for a moment and take inventory of your own life. Are you taking on more than is healthy? Is your stress level balanced or does it lean more toward the bad type of stress? Until you actually stop and look at your life, you may think, as I did, that your stress isn't impacting you physically. You may discover it is, so take a stress inventory for both you and your loved ones.

Mental (brain)

The mental dimension includes various activities to keep your brain active, such as reading, writing, problem solving, and learning new skills. The key to keeping this dimension healthy is exercising the brain through continuous lifelong learning. Embrace the opportunity to read a parenting book, or learn something new at work, for example. You'll be less stressed if you keep up with current techniques, which helps the physical dimension, and you'll be helping the mental dimension as well.

A passion I developed during my cancer recovery was reading books, particularly personal development books. I've read at least thirty of these books since my cancer, and I am convinced I have been better able to control my happiness and success in life by applying the advice they provide.

Another way I keep my brain engaged is by playing brain teaser games such as Sudoku and puzzles. They're fun, yet keep me working on my mental development.

You'll find your own way to stimulate your brain and work in the mental dimension as you take care of yourself. You might want to start with something easy like day dreaming. Think about your ideal life and what that would be like. Or maybe you want to take a class on a topic that you're interested in. Exploring a new hobby or learning a new skill all add to working on the mental dimension of taking care of yourself.

Emotional (heart)

The emotional dimension is all about having meaningful activities and relationships in your life. Your activities can be work-related, volunteer opportunities or ones you do by yourself for others. I know one cancer survivor who enjoys crocheting, then gives her projects away to others.

During my cancer journey, the primary way I met this dimension was by hosting the Shoot for the Cure fundraisers. These experiences kept me surrounded by loads of positive people on a regular basis. Other activities I did to enrich this dimension was become a cancer peer support person to help other breast cancer patients get through their journeys. Then, when I returned to work, I spearheaded a wellness challenge and walking club with colleagues. Any activity I could do or relationship that I could build to help others was emotionally fulfilling.

Take inventory of the activities and relationships in your life. Are they meaningful, satisfying and fulfilling? Do they provide you with positive emotional energy? Consider dropping any that do not meet these criteria so you have more time and energy to spend on the favorable activities and relationships. And if you don't have enough meaningful activities and relationships to fill your emotional needs, this is your time to start exploring new opportunities. The world awaits you.

Spiritual (soul)

The spiritual dimension involves reflecting on your values and purpose in life to ultimately achieve a state of inner peace. Life is a spiritual journey and looking after your soul, the spiritual side of your body, is vitally important.

You have many options for taking care of your spiritual dimension. There are formal religious communities to help you if you're looking for guidance. There's prayer if you want a quiet, personal, spiritual experience. You can try meditation, listening to music, or taking a walk in nature to reflect on your values in life. As you travel your spiritual journey, your life purpose will be revealed to you.

For me, my cancer journey prompted me to spend a lot of time reflecting on my life and trying to determine why we experienced the cancer hat trick. I wondered what message about life I wasn't getting from up above. Pondering this prompted me to read the books I mentioned earlier. I'm still on my spiritual journey, and probably always will be, but I'm living my life with purpose and inner peace more than I did before cancer, and it's wonderful.

The spiritual dimension for each of us is perhaps the most personal of the four dimensions. Reflect on your values, your religious beliefs, and whatever else feeds your soul. Give yourself permission to meditate, to ponder, to process, and to discover your life purpose so you can enjoy inner peace. Getting in touch with your spiritual dimension will enable you to live your life to the fullest.

The cancer statistics provided earlier are sobering, so if there's anything I can do to reduce the chances of cancer coming back, I'm going to do it. I'm resolved to ensure I work on all four dimensions every day, and I hope you are too.

I encourage you to complete the wellness challenge in the appendix, *Your Action Guide*, to see where you can potentially improve.

Chapter Five
Live Your Ideal Life

The Law of Attraction is one of those rules in life that has been spoken about for many years by many different authors. According to author Brian Tracy, the basic principle of the Law of Attraction is that you are a living magnet, attracting into your life the people, situations, and circumstances that are in harmony with your dominant thoughts. I agree completely with this theory, as validated during my cancer journey. This lesson will illustrate how I attracted and achieved my ideal life.

Know What You Want in Life

Have you taken the time recently to really know what makes you happy in life? And know what you really want with clarity? Often this happens when you are faced with a tragedy or health issue (or mid-life crisis hits), but ideally it is done proactively as well. This first step is very important, because if you don't know what makes you truly happy, you won't have a compass to help keep you on track when life throws you challenges. And it works in all situations— attracting an ideal mate, an ideal job, a healthy body, etc.

Determining my purpose in life and what makes me happy was the first key step in my journey to answer the questions—*Why? Why did my family get struck with cancer three times in six months? What message was I just not getting from above?* I used several techniques to help me answer these questions including determining my principles, priorities, passions, personal responsibilities, and ultimately, my ideal life. This was not an easy task and took several months of revisions until I finally determined what I wanted in life.

Personal principles or values are your fundamental beliefs that guide you in your life. If they are not met or being followed, they will often cause you stress.

I identified my personal principles and values as *family comes first, living a balanced life, trying your hardest, and helping others.*

Passions are extraordinary enthusiasm. To enhance our happiness, we should spend as much time as possible on our passions each day. Ideally your work would be your passion, but if not, ensure you find ways to spend other time during the day on your passions.

To help identify my passions, I came up with these questions, and I've included my answers:

- If anything were possible, what would you do? *Have more time and fun with my family; help my husband with his company during the day versus nights and weekends; travel with my family/friends while spreading my inspirational word to help others; host wellness retreats at the cottage.*

- When are you at your happiest? *When I am healthy, content, feeling peaceful, at the cottage, reading personal development books, getting exercise, enjoying a happy family and good family relations.*

- When are you most energized? *When giving speeches and hosting wellness seminars/workshops.*

- What do you care enough about to do for free? *Read and summarize personal development books; help others learn how to be happier on a daily basis; host wellness retreats at my cottage.*

- What activities do you get so absorbed in that you lose track of time? *Watching my kids play hockey, personal development reading, speaking engagements.*

- If you had an opportunity to take any training, what would it be? *Personal development and wellness training.*

- What fills your spirit? *Helping others; time to be there for my family, kids, and raising them well.*

- What are your unique gifts, abilities, and talents? *Inspiring others, being grounded in my principles, enthusiasm, work ethic, leader.*

- What are your personal experiences that have shaped you? *Getting cancer, being a mom, working in management, fundraising, playing sports (hockey and ringette).*

- If you could change one thing in your life, what would it be? *More time spent at a relaxing pace with family and, helping others.*

Personal responsibilities are key roles. Everyone has someone or something that relies on them. Take time to identify your key roles in life that require your time. This is not only helpful when determining your ideal life, but also when helping to prioritize your schedule each week.

My key roles include *myself, my family (kids, spouse, parents), home/cottage owner, work, friends, and community.*

Priorities are also important. To help you stay focused in life and make good decisions, you need to know what your high level priorities are.

Every week, I identify one to three key activities per role, and then schedule them into the calendar to ensure they get done. If you focus on your most important priorities first, the others will fall into place.

Here are some questions for determining your priorities.

- If a loved one was diagnosed with an illness or suffered a tragedy, what regrets, if any, would you have about how you've been spending your time? *I'd spend less time sweating the small stuff or petty issues in our family life.*

- If you knew with certainty that you were going to die in one year, what changes in your life would you make? *This answer may change from time to time. Before I left work, I would have said—spend more time with family at a slower pace. Since leaving work, I am completely at peace with my life.*

- What are the top three to five items on your bucket list[1]? *When I left work, my bucket list items were to write a book, travel with family while doing speaking engagements, and raise a quarter-million dollars for cancer research. It is very gratifying seeing the progress towards achieving these items.*

---

1 *The Bucket List* is a 2007 movie about two terminally-ill men and their wish list of things they'd like to do before they "kick the bucket." The term "bucket list" became a part of popular culture almost immediately upon the film's release.

- What are your top three to five priorities in life? *My health, my family, our family business, my passions.*

Thinking about your answers to the above questions, imagine your ideal life in the following areas, with as much detail as possible. Who would you be with? How would you feel? What would you be doing? Where would you be? I've provided sample answers below based on my life. See the appendix, *Your Action Guide*, to document your answers.

Life—*Feeling peaceful; enjoying fantastic relationships with my family and friends; enjoying excellent health—energized, healthy, vibrant, and excited about each day; helping others—leading, mentoring, inspiring; feeling freedom.*

Family—*Being helpful, contributing, respectful, responsible, confident, fun, happy; looking forward to coming home; home is filled with laughter; enjoying peaceful relations—everyone has patience and self-awareness to handle all issues in an appropriate calm manner; being the best we can be; living in a beautiful home and cottage; giving back to society.*

Relationship—*Someone who makes me laugh; is patient and a good listener; enjoys travelling, going to a cottage, social activities; values me as an equal—asks for my input into decision-making; shares the household duties.*

Financial Situation—*Enough money to easily pay the bills and save for the future; enough money to share with others; enough money for a happy retirement.*

Health—*Getting exercise every day by following my workout videos; riding my bike; going for walk/jogs with my friends; kayaking, biking, swimming, and walking/jogging at the lake; eating healthy every day; being at my ideal weight; feeling energized; taking time to renew myself on all four dimensions every day.*

Focus on What You Want

To achieve your ideal life, the second step is to spend time and energy on what you have identified as your ideal life. There are many tools to help you accomplish this, including visualization, affirmations, meditation, and making good choices.

Visualization

Visualization is a mental technique used by athletes, actors, and other successful people all the time. You use your imagination to see your dreams and make them come true. This works because the brain does not differentiate between what is imagined and what is real. If you visualize something specific, you can attract that something to you. The size of the something isn't what's important here. The power of the visualization is what counts.

Start the visualization process by closing your eyes and, using as many of the five senses as you can. Imagine whatever it is you dream of—healthy body, specific job, etc. See yourself attaining your dream. The more you see what you want, the more you'll feel it. The more you feel it, the more attention you'll give it and the faster you'll receive it.

You can enhance the power of visualizations by creating cue cards of your ideal vision and posting them around the house/office (bathroom, fridge, computer, car, desk etc.). You can also create a photo/picture collage of your ideal vision.

I used this technique frequently when going through my cancer treatments to help me visualize my healthy cancer-free body, and continue using it to visualize my ideal life and family.

Affirmations

Affirmations are powerful words or phrases for improving your life. They describe something and, when repeated over and over, settle in the subconscious mind and manifest themselves in positive action. You need more than simple repetition, however. You also need conviction and desire. You need to want whatever it is the affirmation is about. Remember, you attract into life what is in harmony with your dominant thoughts. So repeating your desires helps make these your dominant thoughts, thus attracting them sooner.

Good affirmations are short, specific, empowering, and use present tense, as if whatever you're affirming is current.

Here are some affirmations you may want to try.

- I love my life and my healthy body.
- I am beating my cancer hands down.
- I am enjoying a happy relationship with my family.
- I am acing this job interview (or meeting) today.
- I love my job and look forward to getting to the office every day.
- I feel great today.
- Today is a terrific day.
- Life is wonderful.

Affirmations were another tremendous technique for helping me remain positive through my journey, and attracting my ideal life. Try affirmations and feel the positive power in your life too.

Meditation

Meditation is a technique that utilizes the power of the subconscious mind to connect with God, a Higher Power, or the Universe—depending on your spiritual beliefs. It comes in many varieties and there are a variety of practitioners who can teach you to meditate. Or you can learn more about meditations through books or the Internet. In general, meditation is an internal practice wherein you relax and focus on a specific image, word or sound, such as your breathing or ideal vision.

I used this technique during my cancer treatments usually once a day to relax and restore my positive energies and allow me to focus on my ideal vision—beating the cancer. I continue to use it on a regular basis to relax and focus on my ideal life.

Choice

Many people have a hard time saying no as well as making decisions. The simplest formula when faced with a decision in life is to decide whether or not the decision will take you closer to your ideal vision or further away. If closer, then consider it. If further, then learn to say no.

For example, I used to think that every opportunity to

participate in an activity was important and I would try to fit them all into my life. Until I realized it was making me way too busy and unhappy. Now that I know my health, my family, and a slower pace of life are my priorities, it is easier to make decisions and say no when necessary.

Another area that many people struggle with making choices about is career. What education should you take? What career should you strive for? Which job opportunity should you take? Do you want to work full time, part time, or not at all? Do you need to stay working, or can you quit or retire early? These are all very good questions with no single answer. However, do remember that in most situations, you are in control. You do have a choice.

For example, if you don't like your job, you can always look for another one. Yes, it may be difficult, or you may be reluctant to give up your current benefits or pay cheque, but you do have a choice. And the fact you are in control of this choice is a very empowering feeling.

The key is to keep focused on what your ideal vision is, and then make choices that move you closer to this vision.

Perhaps you're a working parent who is living a hectic life. Many times you feel like you do not have a choice — you have to work to provide for the family. And you may be right in that you do need to work. But the question is do you really need to work in the specific job you have if it is not meeting your ideal vision or your principles and priorities. No.

First make sure you have a clear vision of your ideal life and your principles and priorities. For me, it was a more balanced life at a slower pace.

Next, evaluate your current job against this ideal. If it's in harmony, then no changes are required. However, if your life is not in harmony with your principles and ideal vision, then determine what changes are needed.
Based on your financial situation, you may need to stay working, but perhaps you can find ways to alter your current job or look for a different job that will better meet your principles and needs. Or, you can consider switching to part time work to better meet your ideal life. Or, perhaps you can "retire" from your job completely.

While these are all valid choices, often people think they have no options, where in reality they do. It just comes down to priorities. For example, do you need a new car, or could you survive with a used car? Do you need the size of house you have in your current neighborhood, or is it more of a luxury versus necessity?

If reducing stress by working less hours or in a position making less money is more important than your material needs and wants, then you can choose to make changes. Or, you can choose to stay at your job, because it provides you with a closer vision to your ideal life. It's up to you. Just listen to your heart and stay true to your principles and priorities.

To achieve your ideal life, you need to focus on what you want every day. Skip a day and it's easy to lose the momentum. Whichever tools you use to focus on what you want in life, you need to stay true to your principles, passions, and priorities. This prepares you for the final step in this lesson—getting what you want.

Get What You Want in Life

This is the last step in Living Your Ideal Life. Now that you are paying attention and focusing on what you want, you need to allow it into your life. By that I mean don't stress about it and don't limit yourself by thinking there is only one way to reach your goal. If you limit yourself, you won't see all the other opportunities that appear in your life to help you. Be open to what appears around you.

I've learned and grown the most in this step, both during and following my cancer journey. Getting what you want is all about removing any doubt about your desires and instead, spending your energy on gratitude and appreciating each day of life. It's also about relaxing and enjoying the journey while you allow answers to unfold around you regarding your life's desires.

I used to be very driven and always wanting to be in control of my life. This turned out to be very problematic with my cancer diagnosis and journey since I had no control over the diagnosis, timing of surgery, treatment delays due to low blood counts, etc.

I had to learn to accept the things I could not control. I learned how to relax and trust God's plan and to be happy with life the way it was. Those lessons benefitted me not only in surviving my cancer, but also in dealing with other life issues, including my teenage boys and my career.

Regarding my career, I thought I had to stay at work to maintain family financial stability. Then one day I did an analysis and discovered I really didn't have to stay at work. I had a desire to slow down the pace of life to achieve better balance, to spend more time with my family, to share my inspirational insights with others facing major health issues or other life-altering situations and I could do it after all. What a joyful day that was.

You can get what you want in life too. Following are some great techniques I used in this step.

Live Your Ideal Life

Appreciation and gratitude. Take time to appreciate anything. It's the feeling that's attached to your appreciation that's important, because it's the feeling that helps send out the strong positive vibrations. Try saying something grateful to a family member or sending an appreciative note to a colleague or even writing about what you're grateful for in a journal on a daily basis.

Read books that inspire you to become your best self. I have many, but there's a series that helped me and it begins with *Don't Sweat the Small Stuff* by Richard Carlson. He offers short lessons about how to relax in life and enhance your positive vibrations, and thus, your ultimate happiness. Whichever book (or series of books) you choose, reading them and applying the concepts should help you achieve your ideal life.

Enjoy the journey. By this I mean keep your goal and vision of what you want in front of you, then learn to enjoy each day as you make your way through life. Of course, goals are important, but if you postpone all your happiness for when you achieve the goal, your happiness will be short-lived. Enjoying the journey along the way will help increase (and extend) your happiness levels. I used to be so driven by my never-ending to-do list as I

---

2 Carlson, Richard. *Don't Sweat the Small Stuff*. New York: Hyperion, 1996.

raced through life trying to get everything done that I forgot to enjoy each activity on the list. I missed out on so much. Now I take time to appreciate each activity, and I plan at least one joyful endeavor per day. It could be a family activity, a massage, or ten minutes reading a good book in a warm bubble bath. The key is to consciously think about what you're looking forward to every day to enhance your positive feelings.

Mindfulness. This is the state of being attentive to and aware of what is going on in the present moment—no judgment, evaluation, or reaction—just awareness. We often spend much of our time reliving the past or fretting about the future. When we do that, we tend to miss the only time we actually have—the present. Think about how many times you've driven to work and you remember leaving your house and arriving at work, but everything in between is a blank—you made the journey, but were unaware of anything connected with it because you were somewhere else in your consciousness. Next time you're driving to work, be mindful of your surroundings and appreciate the brightness of the sun, the beauty of the trees and flowers, the abundant display of wealth (cars, homes, etc.), and the interesting people you see. You'll notice things that have always been there, but you just missed them. Be present, feel less stress and see life anew.

Balance. Racing from place to place is a good indicator something's out of balance in your life. Before cancer, I lived a hectic lifestyle. I raced from work to home to kids' activities and forgot about me in the process. Granted, all of what I just listed may need to happen, but they could have happened at a slower pace. Create balance by slowing down and allowing others to help you. Do you really need that extra promotion that will just take up more of your time? Can some of the housework duties be delegated, hired out, or simply standards relaxed? And while we all want to be super parents, do your kids really need to be in every activity possible at the same time? Take time to focus on your goals and desires and appreciate each day and your loved ones around you.

Relax and trust God's plan. This is an ongoing process. I really do believe that everything happens for a reason and when the timing is right, the answers will become clear. When I was in what I call my "research" phase—the phase where I was exploring what I should be doing with the rest of my life after cancer, I pondered many options, including whether or not to return to work. Eventually I learned how to let go of the how and when and trust that God would provide those answers when the timing was right. When I set my personal life vision to spend more time with my family while working to help others see the potential for their own lives, I had no idea how that could ever be possible. And now I'm living it. I just had to relax and trust God's plan for me.

Do each of the three steps to this lesson and you'll see they work. I spent lots of time on step one, knowing what you want, when I was having chemo treatments and was off work for a year. The following two years I focused on my ideal life and being happy on a daily basis. Then, in year three, I finally got what I wanted when I made the decision to leave my corporate job to better align with my principles, priorities, and passions.

Your journey may be different, the timing may change for you. You may not need to leave your job to achieve your ideal life. But when you live in harmony with your principles, priorities, and passions, you can increase your happiness—even in the face of adversity.

Chapter Six
Daily Happiness Check List

While the steps described in the last three chapters are the key steps to improving your happiness and success in life in the long run, I learned it was also important to create a check list to follow on a daily basis to help keep you on track and happy in the short term.

This list is especially important to keep you positive and focused while you are still in the process of achieving your ideal life, as well as on days when you're stressed or feeling blue.

The key to this check list is to:

1. Create a list of things that you can control on a daily basis that are important to your happiness.
2. Ensure you personalize it to what's meaningful in your life and what helps you to be happy on a daily basis.
3. Perform the steps on a daily basis, referring to the check list as often as necessary.

4. Vary the actual activities within each step to prevent boredom.

Here is my daily happiness check list.

1. Begin and end each day with positive reflection, such as:

    a. Prayer.

    b. Appreciation and gratitude.

    c. Vision statement and affirmations.

    d. Trusting God's plan.

2. Plan at least one activity per day that you're looking forward to, then consciously think about it during the day.

3. Exercise daily—take care of yourself first in all four dimensions.

4. Be present—take time to enjoy your family, colleagues, friends, and each event that happens in your day.

5. Perform an act of kindness.

What is your daily happiness check list?

PART THREE

Epilogue

Chapter Seven
Live Your Life to the Fullest

My journey is living proof that you can survive adversity and be happier. Living your life to the fullest is possible. The ultimate test goes back to the question—should you be told with certainty that you will die in a year, would you make changes? For the first time in my life, I can honestly say that I am totally at peace with my life. I would not make any significant changes should I find out my cancer is back, I may die in a year, or a loved one is diagnosed with an illness. Now my challenge is to maintain this peaceful state.

And while I don't know exactly what the future will look like, for once I am not scared by that uncertainty. Rather I am energized by the opportunities that lie ahead. And peaceful knowing that should my cancer come back, I've done everything possible to ensure I'll have no regrets—I'm living my life based on my principles, priorities and passions. I can't ask for anything more.

For me, living my life to the fullest includes:

- Thinking positively and being happy on a daily basis.
- Taking care of myself first, including balance in my life.
- Taking time to appreciate life, family and friends and to be more present with them.
- Pursuing my dreams and passions (even if part time).
- Finding ways to give back to society, such as organizing and supporting cancer fundraisers.

Now it's your turn to live your life to the fullest. I challenge you to embrace the lessons in this book. Beginning today, how will you spend your time and what decisions will you make that will allow you to have no regrets in your final hours? In other words, how will you live your life to its fullest, starting today?

Your imagination and determination are the only things holding you back from ensuring you are living your life to its fullest. And you don't need to change everything overnight. One step at a time is all that's needed to make positive changes. You can take steps now toward living your ideal life with no regrets. The great news is you're in control. Start with one small step today, then keep your commitment to yourself and remember to hold yourself accountable for your progress. Living life to its fullest is so worth it!

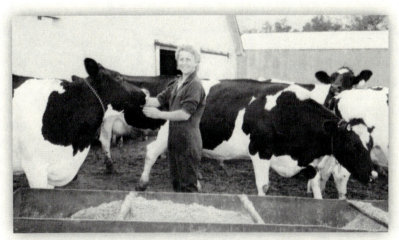

Growing up on a dairy farm taught me the value of hard work and positive thinking.

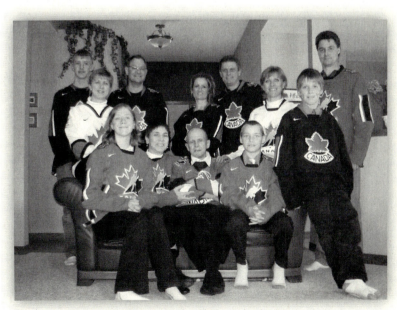

My entire family loves hockey!

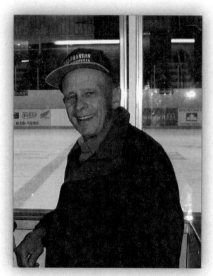

My dad Connie Bossuyt at the rink — watching 11 hockey games in one weekend was his record!

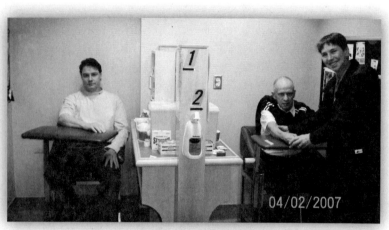

Darryl's first chemo treatment coincided with Dad's biopsy appointment at the same hospital.

Cancer Scores a Hat Trick

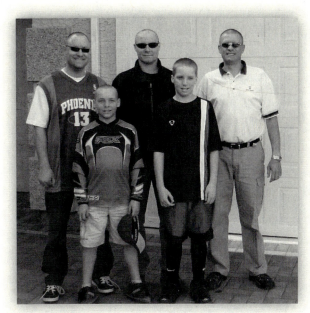

My family showed their support for Darryl during his chemo treatments by shaving their heads.

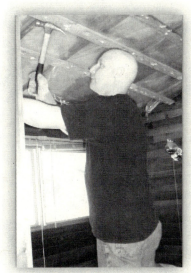

Working on the cottage renovations gave Darryl something positive to focus on during his chemo treatments.

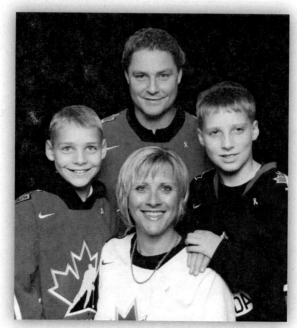

A portrait of our family taken just before I started chemo treatments.

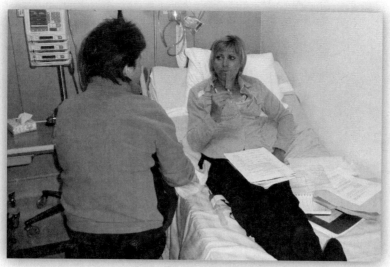

Sucking on popsicles during chemo treatments helped prevent mouth blisters.

Cancer Scores a Hat Trick

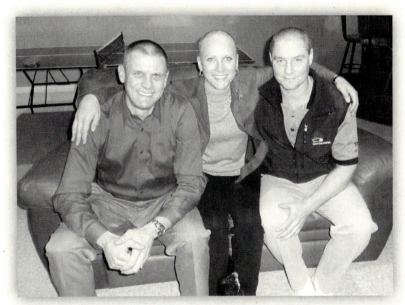

Christmas 2008. I had lost my hair from chemo treatments and my brother Randy and husband Darryl shaved theirs.

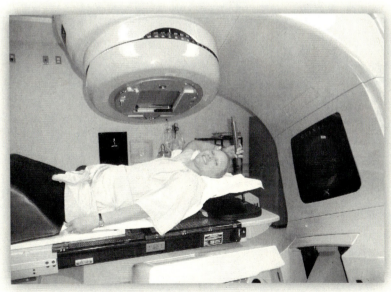

I went for daily radiation treatments for six weeks.

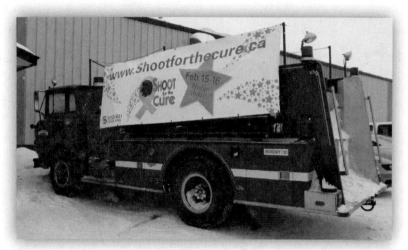

The whole community got behind the "Shoot for the Cure" fundraiser.

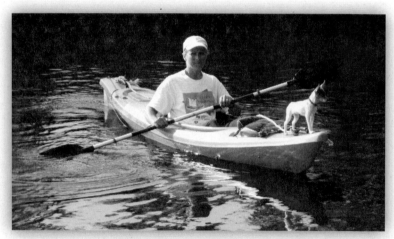

Enjoying time at my cottage kayaking with our dog Sidney.

Cancer Scores a Hat Trick

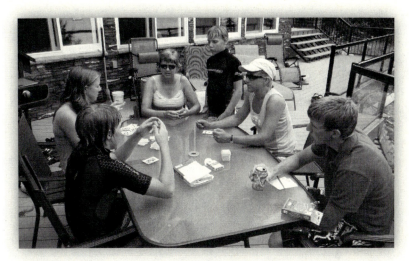

During my cancer year, summer at the lake with the family was one of the best times of my life.

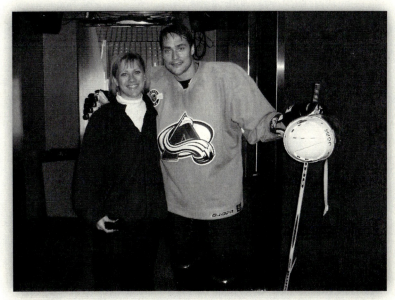

In 2004, I met Teemu Selanne, my family's hockey idol from the former Winnipeg Jets.

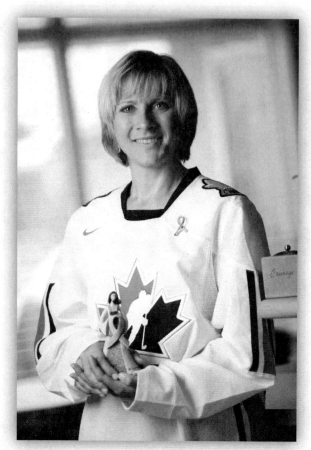

With our hat trick diagnosis, hockey and cancer became inextricably linked for our family. I'm holding a 'cancer angel' in this photo taken just before I started chemo treatments.

Appendix

Your Action Guide

It's wonderful you've come this far reading this book. You've read my family's story in facing cancer's hat trick. You've learned the lessons of positive thinking, taking care of yourself first, and living your ideal life. You've probably even embraced the concept of living life to its fullest. But how do you put it into action? Simple. Take some time to complete this action guide so you can ensure you are happy, healthy, and living your life to the fullest. Remember, though, this is a life-altering tool and not just a quick fix. It took me several months to determine, and then several years to achieve, my ideal life. But the time and effort are worth it. Take your time, reflect on your answers, follow the steps, and eventually you will achieve success too.

The Power of Positive Thinking

Thinking positive is not 100 percent instant magic. You may not always get what you hope for or think about. Life hands out challenges all the time. But facing those challenges with positive thoughts enhances your ability to deal with those challenges and to get the outcomes you want.

Coping Techniques to Enhance your Positive Thinking

- Determine the worst case scenario, decide how you would handle it, then focus on the best case scenario.
- Look for the silver lining in every situation.
- Focus on the glass being half full, not half empty.
- Find something positive to focus on.
- Surround yourself with positive people.
- Look for the lessons to be learned from every situation.
- Be grateful.
- Perform an act of kindness.
- Read books that inspire you.

Think of a recent challenge you've had to overcome. What coping techniques did you use?

_____
_____
_____
_____

Think of a current challenge you're facing. What coping techniques can you use?

_____
_____
_____
_____

Remember positive thinking takes practise, but it will be well worth it as you learn how to think more positively and to handle life's challenges more peacefully. Some experts suggest 40 percent of your happiness is determined by your intentional activity (attitude and behaviour), so make that activity positive.

Take Care of Yourself First

Almost half of this book's readers will develop cancer at some point in their lives. The good news is the survival rates are increasing every day and over half of all cancers can be avoided by introducing fundamental changes to your lifestyle and by taking care of yourself first.

Remember the four key dimensions to taking care of yourself — physical, mental, emotional, spiritual. If it's easier, you may want to think body, brain, heart, soul. That works too.

To help you better understand some potential renewal activities in each of these dimensions, I've included a sample wellness challenge score card below. I encourage you to fill this out and see where you can improve. To complete it, simply:

1. Review the activity listing, using the blank rows to add in any additional wellness activities that are important to you.

2. Score yourself for yesterday in column Y (one point if activity performed).

3. Score yourself for the next week (days 1-7) and see how much improvement you can make.

4. Pick one or two activities that you want to work on for twenty-one days to make it a habit.

Wellness Challenge Score Card

Activity	Y	1	2	3	4	5	6	7
1. Physical								
Eat 7-10 servings of fruits and vegetables daily								
Drink 6-8 glasses of water daily								
Drink 2 glasses of water as soon as you get up								
Eat a healthy breakfast								
Get away from your desk every lunch hour								
Take stretch breaks								
30 minutes of moderate to vigorous endurance activity.								
30 minutes of flexibility activity								
30 minutes of strength activity								
Have a nap during the day								
7-9 hours of sleep each night								

Appendix

Activity	Y	1	2	3	4	5	6	7
2. Mental								
Play a brain game (e.g. Sudoku, crossword puzzle)								
Play a board game								
Play a memorization game								
Read a book								
Engage in a creative endeavor								
Read the newspaper/watch the news								
Learn something new								
3. Emotional								
Positive self-talk								
Smile and laugh								
Listen to music								
Relaxation breathing								
Pamper yourself								
Spend time with a friend								
Perform a random act of kindness								
Make a new friend								
Volunteer								
Attend a social gathering								

Activity	Y	1	2	3	4	5	6	7
4. Spiritual								
Positive self-reflection or affirmation								
Meditate								
Practice yoga								
Practice Tai Chi								
Read/write something inspirational								
Express gratitude								
Journal								
Connect with nature								
Read something spiritual								
Scores								

Know What You Want in Life

To ensure you are happy, healthy, and living your life to the fullest, you need to know what it is that you want and makes you happy—your *ideal life*. The following questions will provide you with details for the concluding *ideal* exercise.

Personal principles or values are your fundamental beliefs that guide you in your life. What are your personal principles or values that guide you? Remember, yours will be unique to you.

Appendix

_____

_____

_____

_____

Passions—To enhance your happiness, you should spend as much time as possible each day on activities that provide you satisfaction while losing track of time. So what are your passions? Answer these questions to help determine your passions.

If anything were possible, what would you do?

_____

_____

_____

_____

When are you at your happiest?

_____

_____

_____

When are you most energized?

_____

What do you care enough about to do for free?

What activities do you get so absorbed in that you lose track of time?

If you had an opportunity to take any training, what would it be?

Appendix

What fills your spirit?

_____

_____

_____

_____

What are your unique gifts, abilities and talents?

_____

_____

_____

_____

What are your personal experiences that have shaped you?

_____

_____

_____

_____

If you could change one thing in your life, what would it be and why?

_____

_____

_____

_____

Personal responsibilities—Everyone has someone or something that relies on them. Take time to identify your key roles in life that require your time. This is not only helpful when determining your ideal life, but also when helping to prioritize your schedule each week.

What are your key roles?

_____

_____

_____

_____

Priorities—To help you stay focused in life, you need to know what your high level priorities are. Answer these questions to help determine your priorities.

If a loved one was diagnosed with an illness or suffered a tragedy, what regrets, if any, would you have about how you've been spending your time?

_____

_____

_____

_____

Appendix

If you knew with certainty that you were going to die in one year, what changes in your life, if any, would you make?

_____
_____
_____
_____

What are the top three to five items on your bucket list?

_____
_____
_____
_____

What are your top three to five priorities in life?

_____
_____
_____
_____

Ideal Life—Thinking about your answers to the above questions, imagine your ideal life in the following areas, with as much detail as possible. Who would you be with? How would you feel? What would you be doing? Where would you be? Tip: To help think of additional details, think of what you do *not want*, and then the opposite is what you do want.

Life (your life overall)

_____

_____

_____

_____

Family

_____

_____

_____

_____

Relationship

_____

_____

_____

_____

Financial Situation

_____

_____

Appendix

_____

_____

Health

_____

_____

_____

Career

_____

_____

_____

Focus On What You Want

Once you know what you want in life, you need to focus on it. You can think about, even write down what you want, but to achieve it requires focus—creating an environment and mindset that allows you to get the people and circumstances into your life that will help you achieve what you want.

Here are some techniques to help you focus on your ideal life.

Visualization

- Start the visualization process by closing your eyes and,

using as many of the five senses as you can, imagine whatever it is you dream of—healthy body, specific job, etc. See yourself attaining whatever your dream is. The more you see *what* you want, the more you'll feel it. The more you feel it, the more attention you'll give it and the faster you'll receive it.

- Create cue cards of your ideal life, family, relationship, financial situation, health and/or career and post them around the house/office. Suggested places are in the bathroom, on the fridge, on your computer screen, in your car, at your desk, etc.

- Create a vision board (photo/picture collage) of your ideal life, family, relationship, financial situation, health and/or career.

Affirmations

An affirmation is a word or phrase you say repeatedly to yourself on any subject or thought. Good affirmations are short, specific, empowering, and use the present tense. Choose from the sample list provided or create some new affirmations of your own to support your ideal life, family, relationship, financial situation, health and/or career.

Sample Affirmations

General
- There is so much joy in my life.

- I like myself, I really like myself.
- I am a wonderful, caring, giving person.
- Something wonderful is happening to me today.
- I am successful at anything I set my mind to.
- Everywhere I look, new opportunities present themselves.
- Success comes naturally for me.
- Every day in every way—I'm getting better and better.

Health
- I am a healthy person—physically, mentally, emotionally and spiritually.
- I feel terrific. I feel great.
- I am acing this next chemo treatment.
- I am beating this cancer hands down.
- I am getting exercise at least five times per week.
- I am promoting healthy eating at every opportunity.

Career/School
- I love knowing I inspire people.
- I love my job and look forward to getting to the office every day.
- I am confident, relaxed and ready to ace this interview/presentation/test.

Family
- I'm a wonderful parent.
- I love being with my happy, healthy, and helpful family.

Spouse
- I'm a wonderful spouse.
- I have a loving and supportive spouse and healthy relationship.

Friends
- I have many great friends and colleagues.
- My friends and colleagues all have good intentions.

Your Affirmations

_____

_____

_____

_____

Meditation

There are many different types of meditation, including guided mantra, loving kindness, sleep relaxation, stress release, body scan, spiritual/prayer, compassion/happiness, imagery scripts, counting, affirmations, etc.

There are numerous meditation and relaxation exercises available in cds, books, and online. Do a Google search on "free meditation scripts" and explore the many techniques and samples provided. Then save your favorites, so that you can refer to them anytime to read or listen to, including on a coffee break at work. Or print them off if you prefer.

Appendix

Using these resources, I created the following exercise for my own use and you may find it helpful for you. If you'd like to create your own, do an Internet search for custom meditation or relaxation scripts and you'll find many resources to help you.

Ideal Life Meditation

Begin by finding a comfortable position, seated or lying down. Prepare to relax.

Take a deep breath in, and as you exhale, allow your body to begin to relax.

Breathe slowly and comfortably.

If your mind wanders, that's ok, just take notice and gently guide it back to your breathing.

Continue to breathe deeply—slowly—and naturally.

Count down now, from 5 to 1. As you say each number, you become more relaxed.

Let's begin.

5—Your muscles are relaxing—and becoming heavy—sinking into the chair, floor or bed.... whatever you are touching.

4—Your muscles are sinking deeper and deeper—free of tension.

3—Your mind is relaxing—and you may notice your attention drifting—as you become more relaxed.

2 — You are almost completely relaxed now — feeling peaceful and calm.

1 — You are now deeply relaxed.

Now create a picture in your mind of your ideal life. Imagine feeling happy and calm.

Visualize the details of this life. Where would you be? With who? Doing what?

You feel comfortable, safe and at peace with yourself.

Imagine these following affirmations are true for you, right this moment, and enjoy the positive feelings you experience.

I love my ideal life, and the person I am.

I like myself, I really like myself.

I feel confident, happy and at peace.

I accept myself as I am, knowing I am a human being with flaws. I don't have to be perfect.

I am kind to myself on days when I may be feeling down.

I love my ideal life and all the wonderful people who are part of it.

I accept these people for who they are, as they are.

I accept that people are doing the best they can at the very moment.

I love my ideal life and all the activities within it.

I accept any challenges in life as part of my journey.

I enjoy each day fully.

I look forward to the future.

I love my ideal life and the joyful feelings.

I feel peaceful.

I feel content.

I feel happy.

I love my ideal life.

Notice the feelings you are experiencing. Accept these feelings without judgment. Allow yourself to feel at peace, secure and happy about the future.

Continue to enjoy these positive feelings as you return to your day.

It's time now to reawaken your body and mind — gradually becoming more alert.

Count to 5. When you reach 5, you will be fully awake and feeling peaceful and energized.

1 — You are feeling calm.

2 — You are becoming more awake and alert.

3 — You are feeling peaceful.

4 — You are almost completely awake now.

5 — You are feeling full of energy and refreshed.

Choices

Making decisions in life can be difficult as we often have many choices. Make decisions that will take you closer to your ideal life. You can tell if a decision is in favor of your ideal life, as the answer will feel right and less stressful. By learning how to say no to the low value choices, you are actually saying yes to the higher value choices.

Identify an upcoming decision, and then determine which answer will take you closer to your ideal life.

_____

_____

_____

_____

Schedule Your Priorities First

In an earlier exercise, you identified your ideal life in each of your key roles. Now you need to schedule the key priorities of each role into your calendar.

1. Take your key roles from the prior exercise and insert into the first column below.

2. Determine one simple annual goal for this role, then monthly, then weekly.

3. Schedule this weekly activity right into your calendar.

4. Review your weekly calendar at the start of each week.

Appendix

5. Ensure you keep your commitments to these weekly goals.
6. Review your calendar at the end of the week. Feel satisfaction and gratitude in meeting your weekly goal. Then update your weekly goal for the next week and schedule it into the calendar.

Key Roles	Annual Goal	Monthly Goal	Weekly Goal/ Activity
Example – parent	Spend more quality time with kids	Purchase a ping pong table	Play ping pong at least 3 times with kids
Example – Homeowner	Complete house renovations	Select all products	Select flooring and brick
1			
2			
3			
4			
5			
6			
7			

Get What You Want

Now that you know what you want, you're focusing on it, you simply need to relax and allow your ideal life to start happening. Practice these techniques to help you get what you want in life.

Appreciation and Gratitude Journal

Take time each day to express appreciation and gratitude for all the wonderful things in our lives. You can write in a journal, say it to others, or simply reflect to yourself.

I am grateful for:

_____

_____

_____

_____

Read Books that Inspire You to Become Your Best Self

Learning how to not stress about the petty issues in life is critical.

Make a plan to read/listen to one of Richard Carlson's *Don't Sweat the Small Stuff* series of books/audios by _____ (date).

Enjoy the Journey

What is one activity that you have planned in your day today that you are looking forward to? Remember to think about it often throughout the day to increase the positive vibrations.

___

Mindfulness

Mindfulness is simply a way to experience life, moment by moment.

Practice these simple mindful exercises on a daily basis to help reduce your stress by keeping you focused on the present moment. It's best if you start with number one, then select from numbers two through five.

1. Sit or stand quietly. Take a few deep calming breaths.

2. Look around and identify five items that you can see. Then identify five different sounds, five items you can feel, five different smells, and then five tastes (yes, they get harder as you go).

3. Identify at least five different objects, naming them such as chairs, people, tables, poster, paper.

4. Identify five different shapes such as rectangle, square, round, curved, jagged, smooth.

5. Identify at least five different colors.

These exercises can be easily done while driving your car, walking to a meeting, or any time you want help calming your mind and learning how to enjoy the present moment.

Balance – Slow Life Down

Determine what your ideal balance in life is, and then find ways to achieve it. Say no to some activities, reduce multi-tasking, and schedule in some down time for yourself and/or with your family.

What does the ideal balance in my life look like:

_____

_____

_____

_____

What is one area of my life that is overwhelming, and what could I do to slow it down?

_____

_____

_____

_____

Relax and Trust God's Plan

Remind yourself on a daily basis that you are doing exactly

what you are meant to do each moment of the day. If you are not achieving the results you want, it could be because the timing isn't right yet. What can you learn from your current situation?

_____

_____

_____

What is one area of your life that you could benefit by relaxing and trusting God's plan.

_____

_____

_____

Daily Happiness Check List

While the last few steps will help you achieve your desired life in the long term, it is also important to have a personalized daily check list to help enhance your happiness in the short term.

Identify five activities that you can do and control that are important to your daily happiness.

_____

_____

_____

_____

Live Your Life to its Fullest

You are the only one holding you back from living your life to its fullest and with no regrets. Living a life that makes you happy begins with you. Give yourself permission to make the rest of your life the best it can be. You can do it!

Suggested Reading

- *7 Habits of Highly Effective People* – Stephen Covey
- *Law of Attraction* – Michael Losier
- *The Passion Test* – Janet Bray Attwood & Chris Attwood
- *The Purpose Driven Life* – Rick Warren
- *Three Big Questions* – Dave Phillips
- *Don't Sweat the Small Stuff Series: At Work, At Home, In Life, With Family, etc.* – Richard Carlson
- *Happier* – Tal Ben-Shahar
- *The How to of Happiness* – Sonja Lyubomirsky
- *Happy for No Reason* – Marci Shimoff
- *Who Moved My Cheese* – Spencer Johnson
- *Peaks and Valleys* – Spencer Johnson
- *The Present* – Spencer Johnson
- *How Full is Your Bucket* – Tom Rath & Donald Clifton
- *Mastering the Art of Coping in Good Times and Bad* – Linda Edgar

About the Author

As a successful career woman, community activist, avid hockey mom, and dedicated wife, Shawnda Muir lived the good life—or so she thought until 2007, when she came face-to-face with cancer in her family not once, but three times in a few short months. Her husband was the first one diagnosed. Six weeks later, her father was diagnosed. And six months later, Shawnda herself received her own cancer diagnosis.

Shawnda eventually left her corporate job to pursue her purpose and passion—helping others affected by cancer. As a cancer survivor, author, speaker, workshop leader, wellness retreat facilitator, and successful fundraiser, Shawnda has reached thousands with her message. While still undergoing chemotherapy treatments, Shawnda organized a community fundraiser that raised an incredible $135,000 the first year. She has continued to lead this fundraiser annually, reaching nearly a quarter million dollars in the first three years.

Shawnda has a Bachelor of Commerce degree from the University of Manitoba, many years in senior management as well as entrepreneurship. Shawnda grew up in a large family on a grain and dairy farm in Oak Bluff, Manitoba, Canada and draws on those roots daily. She continues to reside in Oak Bluff with her husband, Darryl, and two sons Justin and Devin.

Visit her at her website, www.shawndamuir.com.